Health Benefits of Blackstrap Molasses

Chapter List:

Book Introduction:

In a world that constantly clamors for the latest trends in health and wellness, one natural elixir has quietly stood the test of time, waiting to be rediscovered. Welcome to "Nourishing Secrets: Unveiling the Healing Power of Blackstrap Molasses." Within the pages of this book, you will embark on a journey through history, science, and personal anecdotes, all weaving together to uncover the remarkable health benefits hidden within a humble sweetener.

For centuries, blackstrap molasses has been cherished as a potent remedy, a trusted source of nourishment, and a versatile ingredient in the culinary realm. In this comprehensive guide, we delve deep into the secrets of blackstrap molasses, exploring its rich nutritional profile, its healing properties, and its transformative effects on the mind, body, and soul.

Chapter 1: The Sweet Essence of History
[>1000]

In the first chapter, we travel back in time to unearth the origins of blackstrap molasses. From the ancient civilizations that treasured its natural sweetness to the centuries-old traditions that recognized its medicinal properties, we discover how this remarkable elixir has been revered throughout history.

Step by step, we unravel the fascinating journey of blackstrap molasses, tracing its path from the sugarcane fields of the tropics to the tables of the elite. Along the way, we encounter the artisans who perfected the art of molasses production, and the pioneers who recognized its potential as a natural remedy.

This chapter serves as a foundation, laying the historical groundwork for the subsequent exploration of blackstrap molasses' incredible health benefits. By understanding its roots, we gain a deeper appreciation for the wisdom of our ancestors and the timeless gift they have left behind.

So, join me as we delve into the enchanting world of blackstrap molasses, where history and healing intertwine to create a tapestry of well-being and nourishment. Get ready to unlock the secrets that have been hidden within the sweet depths of this extraordinary elixir. Your journey to a healthier and more vibrant life begins here, with "Nourishing Secrets: Unveiling the Healing Power of Blackstrap Molasses."

Chapter 2: A Spoonful of Nutritional Gold
[>1000]

As you turn the pages of "Nourishing Secrets: Unveiling the Healing Power of Blackstrap Molasses," the essence of this remarkable elixir becomes even more tantalizing. In Chapter 2, we uncover the golden treasure trove of nutritional goodness that blackstrap molasses holds within its dark, velvety depths.

Imagine holding a spoonful of molasses up to the light and witnessing the radiant glow of essential vitamins and minerals. This thick, luscious liquid is an abundant source of iron, calcium, magnesium, potassium, and B vitamins. Each sip or drizzle promises to nourish your body from the inside out, revitalizing your very core.

But it is not just the nutritional content that makes blackstrap molasses truly special. It is the way in which these nutrients are intricately balanced, working synergistically to support your overall well-being. It's as if nature herself designed this elixir with the utmost care, ensuring that every drop holds the key to unlocking your body's full potential.

As you delve deeper into this chapter, you will discover the transformative power of blackstrap molasses on your energy levels. Feel the surge of vitality as the iron within it boosts your red blood cell production, banishing fatigue and revitalizing your every step. Experience the gentle embrace of calcium, fortifying your bones and teeth, empowering you to stand tall and strong. And let the magnesium and potassium sweep through your body, soothing tired muscles, and promoting a sense of calm and balance.

But it doesn't stop there. Blackstrap molasses offers more than just a nutritional boost. It holds an emotional resonance, a reminder of simpler times and the comfort of cherished traditions. Close your eyes and envision generations past, savoring the sweetness of molasses in their favorite family recipes. Let the nostalgia wash over you, connecting you to a collective memory of love, nourishment, and shared experiences.

Within the pages of this chapter, you will find not only scientific insights and nutritional facts but also the emotional and sensory journey that blackstrap molasses invites you to embark upon. Open your heart and allow yourself to be enveloped by the warmth and sweetness that this elixir offers. Let it heal not only your body but also your spirit, as it whispers stories of generations past, reminding you of the power of nature's gifts.

With each passing page, "Nourishing Secrets: Unveiling the Healing Power of Blackstrap Molasses" becomes more than just a guidebook; it becomes a companion, a confidant that walks alongside you on this path to wellness. So, take a moment to savor the anticipation, for the journey has only just begun. Embrace the nourishing secrets that await you, and let blackstrap molasses guide you towards a life filled with vitality, balance, and heartfelt joy.

Chapter 3: Embracing Nature's Medicine Cabinet
[>1000]

In the depths of "Nourishing Secrets: Unveiling the Healing Power of Blackstrap Molasses," lies a profound realization , blackstrap molasses is not just a sweet indulgence; it is nature's very own medicine cabinet, brimming with remedies that have the power to restore and rejuvenate.

Chapter 3 beckons you to open the doors of this extraordinary cabinet and discover the diverse healing properties that blackstrap molasses possesses. As you step inside, a symphony of aromas and colors surrounds you, captivating your senses and igniting a sense of wonder.

The first shelf holds the antidote for common ailments , the natural remedy that gently eases your discomfort and offers relief. Blackstrap molasses, with its rich mineral content and natural sugars, becomes a soothing balm for digestive troubles. Whether it's indigestion, constipation, or bloating, a spoonful of molasses can work wonders, calming your system and bringing balance to your gut.

As you move deeper into the cabinet, you encounter jars filled with dark, viscous liquids , elixirs for your immune system. Blackstrap molasses emerges as a champion of wellness, fortifying your body's defense mechanisms and bolstering your immune response. Its minerals and antioxidants become the warriors that shield you from harm, protecting you from the onslaught of viruses and infections.

But the magic of blackstrap molasses doesn't end there. It extends its healing touch to your skin, radiating beauty and nourishment. As you explore the next shelf, you discover how this elixir can be transformed into luxurious skincare treatments. The gentle caress of molasses on your skin unleashes its hydrating properties, leaving behind a soft, supple glow. It becomes a remedy for acne, dark spots, and dryness, restoring your skin's natural vitality and helping you embrace your true radiance.

Beyond the shelves of physical healing, blackstrap molasses reaches into the depths of your emotional well-being. It becomes a source of solace, a sweet companion that whispers of comfort during times of stress and anxiety. The rich, caramel tones evoke a sense of warmth and reassurance, as if the elixir itself understands your deepest emotions. It reminds you to slow down, savor the sweetness of life, and find moments of joy amidst the chaos.

In this chapter, we invite you to open your heart to the boundless healing potential that blackstrap molasses holds. Let it be your guide as you embrace the wisdom of nature's medicine cabinet. Allow the emotional depth of this elixir to resonate within you, nurturing not only your body but also your soul.

As you continue to explore the pages of "Nourishing Secrets: Unveiling the Healing Power of Blackstrap Molasses," you will unravel the secrets that lie within each chapter, each word a testament to the transformative power of this humble elixir. So, dear reader, embrace the magic that awaits you and let blackstrap molasses be the catalyst for your journey towards holistic well-being.

Chapter 4: Sweetening the Deal: Culinary Delights with Blackstrap Molasses
[>1000]

As you delve into Chapter 4 of "Nourishing Secrets: Unveiling the Healing Power of Blackstrap Molasses," a world of culinary delights unfolds before you. Blackstrap molasses, with its rich, robust flavor, becomes the star ingredient in a symphony of delectable dishes that are sure to tantalize your taste buds and touch your soul.

Imagine the velvety texture of molasses drizzling over fluffy pancakes on a lazy Sunday morning. Feel the warmth that spreads through your body with each decadent bite, as memories of cherished breakfasts from your childhood come flooding back. Blackstrap molasses becomes not just a topping but a source of comfort, binding generations together in a shared love of food and family.

As you turn the page, you discover the savory wonders that blackstrap molasses can bring to your table. Its deep, caramel notes infuse roasted vegetables with a richness that elevates simple dishes to culinary masterpieces. The golden glaze it creates on succulent grilled meats becomes a work of art, as each brushstroke of molasses turns a meal into a sensory experience.

But it is in the realm of desserts that blackstrap molasses truly shines, transforming sweet treats into blissful indulgences. Imagine the first bite of a soft, gingerbread cookie, the taste of molasses mingling with the spiciness of ginger, taking you on a journey of flavors and emotions. In that moment, you are transported to a place of pure happiness, where time seems to stand still, and all that matters is the joy of savoring every morsel.

And let us not forget the rich, velvety allure of molasses in baking , the way it lends its distinct flavor to moist, dark chocolate cakes and tender, molasses-laced muffins. With each bite, you are enveloped in a sense of nostalgia, recalling the comforting embrace of home and the love that goes into every homemade dessert.

In this chapter, the emotional journey intertwines with the culinary one, for food is more than just sustenance; it is a celebration of life and love. Blackstrap molasses becomes the thread that weaves together the fabric of our cherished memories, bringing together family, friends, and loved ones in moments of joy and togetherness.

As you explore the recipes and stories within this chapter, you are invited to create your own culinary masterpieces, infusing each dish with the love and sweetness that blackstrap molasses imparts. Let it be a reminder of the power of simple pleasures, of finding happiness in the small things, and of cherishing the moments that nourish both body and soul.

In "Nourishing Secrets: Unveiling the Healing Power of Blackstrap Molasses," this chapter becomes more than just a collection of recipes; it becomes a celebration of life's flavors and a journey of self-discovery. So, let the aromas of gingerbread and roasted vegetables fill your kitchen, and let the taste of molasses transport you to a place of joy and comfort. Embrace the culinary delights that await you, and let blackstrap molasses sweeten the deal of your life's grand banquet.

Chapter 5: Revitalizing Your Body: Blackstrap Molasses and Energy Boost [>1000]

In the heart of "Nourishing Secrets: Unveiling the Healing Power of Blackstrap Molasses," lies a chapter dedicated to the transformative energy that this elixir brings to your weary body. Chapter 5 reveals the rejuvenating power of blackstrap molasses, as it breathes new life into every cell, awakening your spirit and igniting a flame of vitality within.

Imagine waking up in the morning, feeling the weight of exhaustion on your shoulders. Your body yearns for an energy boost, a ray of sunshine to pierce through the fog. Blackstrap molasses becomes that radiant light, infusing your being with a renewed sense of vigor and vitality.

As you savor the first sip of a revitalizing molasses-spiked smoothie, you feel the surge of energy coursing through your veins. The natural sugars and rich mineral content become the fuel that propels you forward, banishing fatigue and lifting your spirits. It's as if each drop of molasses contains the essence of the sun, infusing your body with warmth and radiance.

But the energy that blackstrap molasses provides goes beyond a temporary jolt. It nurtures a sustainable vitality that carries you through the day, allowing you to tackle challenges with resilience and grace. Its mineral-rich composition nourishes your cells, supporting their optimal functioning and revitalizing your entire being.

This chapter explores the profound effects of blackstrap molasses on your energy levels, shedding light on the scientific mechanisms that underlie its transformative powers. From the iron that boosts your red blood cell production to the B vitamins that enhance your body's energy metabolism, each nutrient works harmoniously to restore and invigorate.

Yet, blackstrap molasses offers more than a physical energy boost. It becomes a catalyst for embracing life's adventures and finding joy in the simplest moments. As you sip on a warm cup of molasses-spiced tea, you feel a gentle awakening of the senses , a reminder to slow down, breathe, and savor the sweetness of existence.

In the emotional landscape, blackstrap molasses becomes the spark that reignites your passions and renews your enthusiasm. It whispers to your soul, encouraging you to embrace your dreams, chase your ambitions, and find fulfillment in the pursuit of your deepest desires. It becomes the elixir that fuels not only your physical energy but also your inner fire, infusing every step you take with purpose and intention.

As you immerse yourself in the pages of this chapter, let the emotional resonance of blackstrap molasses fill you with a sense of empowerment. Allow it to remind you of the boundless energy that resides within, waiting to be unleashed. Embrace the transformative power of this elixir and let it be the catalyst that propels you towards a life of vitality, passion, and unyielding zest.

"Nourishing Secrets: Unveiling the Healing Power of Blackstrap Molasses" beckons you to embrace the revitalizing energy that awaits you. So, dear reader, take a step forward, feel the surge of life coursing through your veins, and let blackstrap molasses become the key that unlocks your boundless potential.

Chapter 6: Blackstrap Molasses and Inner Harmony: Nurturing Mind and Soul
[>1000]

In the enchanting world of "Nourishing Secrets: Unveiling the Healing Power of Blackstrap Molasses," Chapter 6 beckons you to embark on a journey of inner harmony and soulful nourishment. Here, amidst the pages filled with wisdom and heartfelt insights, you discover the profound connection between blackstrap molasses and the nurturing of your mind and soul.

As you immerse yourself in the warm embrace of blackstrap molasses, you begin to sense a gentle shift in your being. It's as if a soothing melody plays softly in the background, guiding you towards a place of tranquility and peace. The minerals and antioxidants within this elixir become the catalysts that harmonize your inner landscape, bringing balance to the chaos of daily life.

Close your eyes for a moment and envision a cup of hot molasses-infused tea cradled between your palms. As you take a slow, deliberate sip, a sense of calm washes over you, grounding you in the present moment. The rich, caramel notes become a sweet reminder to be mindful, to savor each breath, and to find solace in the beauty that surrounds you.

Within the pages of this chapter, you discover the transformative power of blackstrap molasses in nurturing your mental well-being. Its nutrients, such as magnesium and B vitamins, become the building blocks for a healthy brain, promoting cognitive function, and supporting emotional balance. The elixir becomes a gentle companion, accompanying you on your journey of self-discovery and fostering a deep connection with your inner wisdom.

But it goes beyond the physical realm. Blackstrap molasses reaches into the depths of your soul, stirring emotions and inspiring introspection. It becomes a vessel for self-expression, a sweet medium through which you can explore your innermost thoughts and desires. The act of preparing a molasses-infused meal or indulging in a delectable dessert becomes a form of meditation, a sacred ritual that allows you to reconnect with your inner essence.

In this chapter, you will find nourishment for your soul, as blackstrap molasses becomes the conduit for self-care and self-love. Embrace the nurturing properties of this elixir, allowing it to heal wounds, restore balance, and ignite a spark of creativity within you. Let it serve as a gentle reminder to prioritize your well-being, to listen to the whispers of your heart, and to honor your inner journey.

As you turn the pages, you will encounter stories of individuals who have found solace and serenity in the embrace of blackstrap molasses. Their experiences will inspire you to cultivate moments of stillness, to create space for reflection, and to find beauty in the simple pleasures of life. Allow their stories to touch your heart and awaken a sense of profound connection with yourself and the world around you.

"Nourishing Secrets: Unveiling the Healing Power of Blackstrap Molasses" becomes not just a book, but a sacred guide, leading you towards the path of inner harmony and soulful nourishment. So, dear reader, let the transformative essence of blackstrap molasses infuse your life with tranquility, love, and a deep appreciation for the beauty that resides within you. Open your heart to the nurturing embrace of this elixir, and let it become a source of profound healing for your mind, body, and soul.

Chapter 7: Blackstrap Molasses and the Power of Connection: Embracing Community and Unity
[>1000]

In the captivating tapestry of "Nourishing Secrets: Unveiling the Healing Power of Blackstrap Molasses," Chapter 7 unfolds as a testament to the transformative power of connection and community. Within these pages, the remarkable bond between blackstrap molasses and the human spirit is revealed , a bond that transcends borders, cultures, and generations, weaving a vibrant tapestry of unity and togetherness.

Picture a gathering of souls, a table adorned with a spread of culinary delights infused with the warmth of blackstrap molasses. As friends and family gather around, laughter dances in the air, and stories intertwine, forging unbreakable bonds. Blackstrap molasses becomes the sweet thread that connects hearts, uniting individuals in a shared love for nourishment and the joy of breaking bread together.

In this chapter, you will embark on a journey that explores the power of blackstrap molasses to foster connections, both within ourselves and with others. As you delve deeper, you will witness how this elixir becomes a catalyst for meaningful conversations, a bridge that spans differences, and a symbol of unity in an ever-diverse world.

Imagine a moment of shared delight as you pass a jar of molasses-infused cookies to your neighbor. In that exchange, a connection is forged , a moment of shared joy that transcends language and cultural barriers. Through blackstrap molasses, we discover the common threads that bind us all, reminding us of our shared humanity and the beauty that lies in embracing our differences.

Beyond the physical act of sharing meals, blackstrap molasses becomes a catalyst for cultivating compassion and empathy. It encourages us to open our hearts, to extend a helping hand, and to create spaces where everyone feels seen and heard. The richness of its flavor mirrors the richness of the human experience, inviting us to celebrate diversity and honor the stories that shape us.

As you immerse yourself in the stories and experiences within this chapter, you will witness the transformative power of blackstrap molasses in nurturing a sense of belonging and connectedness. You will meet individuals from all walks of life, united by their love for this humble elixir and their commitment to building inclusive communities. Their stories will ignite a flame of inspiration within you, urging you to seek connections, foster understanding, and create a world where all voices are valued.

"Nourishing Secrets: Unveiling the Healing Power of Blackstrap Molasses" becomes more than just a book; it becomes a call to action , an invitation to embrace the power of connection, unity, and love. It implores you to extend a hand, to build bridges, and to celebrate the diverse tapestry of humanity. Let blackstrap molasses be the catalyst for creating spaces of belonging, where each person's story is honored and cherished.

So, dear reader, open your heart wide and allow the transformative power of blackstrap molasses to guide your journey of connection and community. Let it remind you that together, we are stronger, and that by nurturing bonds of love and understanding, we can create a world where unity flourishes and the sweet taste of togetherness is savored by all.

Chapter 8: Blackstrap Molasses and the Dance of Gratitude: Finding Joy in the Simplest Moments
[>1000]

In the captivating narrative of "Nourishing Secrets: Unveiling the Healing Power of Blackstrap Molasses," Chapter 8 unfolds as a heartfelt ode to the transformative dance of gratitude that emerges when we embrace the simple moments of life. Here, amidst the pages filled with warmth and sincerity, you discover the profound connection between blackstrap molasses and the cultivation of joy, contentment, and appreciation.

Close your eyes for a moment and imagine the rich aroma of freshly baked molasses cookies wafting through the air. As you take a bite, the sweet, velvety goodness melts on your tongue, filling your senses with delight. It is in this simple act of savoring a treat that the dance of gratitude begins , a dance that celebrates the abundance of life and the beauty found in the smallest of gestures.

In this chapter, you will embark on a journey that explores how blackstrap molasses becomes a catalyst for gratitude , a gateway to finding joy and contentment in the simplest of moments. As you dive deeper into its essence, you will witness how this elixir intertwines with the fabric of our existence, infusing each day with a sense of wonder and appreciation.

Picture a scene of a family gathered around the dinner table, sharing a wholesome meal infused with the goodness of blackstrap molasses. As conversations flow and laughter fills the room, a profound sense of gratitude permeates the atmosphere. It is in these moments of togetherness, where love is shared and bonds are strengthened, that the true essence of blackstrap molasses shines , a reminder to be present, to cherish the connections that nourish our souls.

Within the pages of this chapter, you will uncover stories of individuals who have discovered the transformative power of gratitude through their encounters with blackstrap molasses. From a farmer's humble appreciation for the land that yields the molasses, to a child's innocent joy upon tasting a molasses-infused dessert, each story resonates with the simple yet profound truth that gratitude has the power to transform lives.

Blackstrap molasses becomes a gentle teacher, guiding us to slow down and embrace the present moment. It urges us to find solace in the ordinary, to pause and witness the beauty that surrounds us , an intricately woven tapestry of nature's gifts and human kindness. The act of adding a dollop of molasses to a steaming cup of tea becomes a mindful ritual , an invitation to pause, reflect, and express gratitude for the warmth and comfort that life offers.

As you immerse yourself in the pages of this chapter, let the dance of gratitude fill your heart. Allow blackstrap molasses to become the catalyst for a shift in perspective, inviting you to seek beauty in the simplest of moments, to appreciate the blessings that often go unnoticed.

Embrace the transformative power of gratitude and let it illuminate your path, guiding you towards a life filled with joy, contentment, and an unwavering appreciation for all that life offers.

"Nourishing Secrets: Unveiling the Healing Power of Blackstrap Molasses" becomes not just a book but a guidebook for cultivating a grateful heart. It beckons you to embark on a journey of self-discovery, where each day becomes an opportunity to dance with gratitude and celebrate the abundance that surrounds you. So, dear reader, let the dance of gratitude begin, and let blackstrap molasses be the melody that accompanies you on this wondrous journey.

Chapter 9: Blackstrap Molasses and the Tapestry of Resilience: Embracing Strength in Adversity
[>1000]

In the pages of "Nourishing Secrets: Unveiling the Healing Power of Blackstrap Molasses," Chapter 9 unravels as a testament to the profound tapestry of resilience that emerges when we embrace the challenges life presents us. Within these heartfelt pages, you will discover the extraordinary connection between blackstrap molasses and the cultivation of inner strength, courage, and unwavering determination.

Imagine a solitary figure standing amidst a field of sugar cane, their hands gently caressing the tall stalks, weathered yet unwavering. It is through the process of extracting blackstrap molasses that the true essence of resilience is brought to life , a testament to the indomitable spirit that thrives even in the face of adversity.

In this chapter, you will embark on a journey that explores the transformative power of blackstrap molasses in nurturing resilience , the unwavering flame that flickers within us during life's darkest moments. As you delve deeper into its essence, you will witness how this humble elixir becomes a beacon of hope, a source of strength that guides us through the storms and empowers us to rise above our challenges.

Close your eyes for a moment and visualize a spoonful of blackstrap molasses, dark and viscous, held in your palm. As you taste its bittersweet richness, a surge of fortitude courses through your veins, reminding you of your inner strength. Blackstrap molasses becomes a metaphor for resilience , a tangible symbol of the transformative power that resides within each of us.

Within the pages of this chapter, you will encounter stories of individuals who have embraced the tapestry of resilience through their encounters with blackstrap molasses. From individuals who have overcome physical ailments to those who have navigated emotional hardships, each story is a testament to the human spirit's capacity to endure and thrive.

Blackstrap molasses becomes a faithful companion, offering nourishment to both body and soul. Its mineral-rich composition becomes a catalyst for fortitude, supporting the body's ability to heal and renew. But it goes beyond the physical; it becomes a reminder that within the depths of our being, there lies an unyielding strength , an unwavering flame that refuses to be extinguished.

As you immerse yourself in the stories and experiences within this chapter, let the tapestry of resilience enfold you. Allow blackstrap molasses to be your ally in times of trial, a reminder that even in the face of adversity, you possess the power to endure and emerge stronger. Embrace the challenges as opportunities for growth, for it is through the fires of life that the true essence of resilience is forged.

"Nourishing Secrets: Unveiling the Healing Power of Blackstrap Molasses" becomes not just a book, but a guidebook for cultivating resilience in the face of life's trials. It urges you to embrace the storms with an unwavering spirit, to harness the power within, and to emerge transformed. So, dear reader, let blackstrap molasses become the catalyst for your own journey of resilience, empowering you to face life's challenges with grace, determination, and an unyielding belief in your own strength.

Chapter 10: Blackstrap Molasses and the Symphony of Renewal: Embracing Transformation and Growth
[>1000]

As we delve deeper into the heartwarming saga of "Nourishing Secrets: Unveiling the Healing Power of Blackstrap Molasses," Chapter 10 unravels as a poignant ode to the symphony of renewal that unfolds when we embrace the art of transformation and growth. Within these soul-stirring pages, you will discover the profound connection between blackstrap molasses and the journey of self-discovery, evolution, and blossoming into our truest selves.

Imagine a seed nestled in the fertile soil, its potential hidden beneath layers of darkness. As it awakens to the touch of sunlight and the gentle caress of raindrops, the seed unfurls into a magnificent blossom , an exquisite testament to the power of transformation and the beauty of growth.

In this chapter, we embark on a journey that explores the transformative power of blackstrap molasses in nurturing renewal , the tender process of shedding old layers and embracing the blossoming of our true selves. As we immerse ourselves in its essence, we witness how this humble elixir becomes a catalyst for metamorphosis , a sweet reminder that change is a natural part of life's grand tapestry.

Picture a warm mug cradled in your hands, the steam rising as you take a sip of blackstrap molasses-infused tea. With each sip, a gentle sense of rejuvenation courses through your veins, like a melodic symphony of renewal. Blackstrap molasses becomes a conductor of change, guiding us through the intricacies of growth with grace and assurance.

Within the pages of this chapter, you will encounter stories of individuals who have embarked on the path of transformation through their encounters with blackstrap molasses. From individuals who have undergone profound life changes to those who have embraced their authentic selves, each story is a testament to the beauty of embracing the journey of renewal.

Blackstrap molasses becomes a companion on the path of self-discovery, supporting us as we shed the old and welcome the new. Its earthy sweetness becomes a reminder that growth often comes from embracing life's contrasts , the bitter and the sweet, the challenges and the triumphs , all essential in the symphony of renewal.

As we surrender to the dance of transformation, blackstrap molasses becomes a source of comfort, offering nourishment not only to our physical bodies but also to our souls. It encourages us to step into the unknown, to embrace vulnerability, and to find solace in the process of becoming.

As you immerse yourself in the stories and experiences within this chapter, let the symphony of rcncwal resonate within you. Allow blackstrap molasses to be your ally on this journey of growth, reminding you that like the seasons, life is an ever-changing tapestry of experiences. Embrace the moments of renewal with open arms, for it is in the dance of transformation that we truly discover our essence.

"Nourishing Secrets: Unveiling the Healing Power of Blackstrap Molasses" becomes more than just a book; it becomes a guidebook for embracing the symphony of renewal in our lives. It urges us to be gentle with ourselves, to embrace the process of growth with patience and kindness. So, dear reader, let blackstrap molasses be the catalyst for your own journey of transformation, inspiring you to blossom into the fullest expression of your true self and find joy in the ever-evolving melody of life.

Chapter 11: Blackstrap Molasses and the Whispers of Healing: Embracing Wellness and Restoration
[>1000]

As we continue our enchanting exploration through the captivating narrative of "Nourishing Secrets: Unveiling the Healing Power of Blackstrap Molasses," Chapter 11 unravels as a tender embrace of the whispers of healing that echo through our beings when we wholeheartedly embrace wellness and restoration. Within these evocative pages, you will uncover the profound connection between blackstrap molasses and the journey toward physical and emotional well-being.

Imagine a gentle breeze caressing your skin, carrying with it the essence of renewal and vitality. It is in these fleeting moments that we catch whispers of healing, inviting us to embark on a journey of restoration , an invitation that blackstrap molasses graciously extends.

In this chapter, we embark on a transformative journey that explores the healing power of blackstrap molasses , the elixir that nurtures our bodies and minds with its rich tapestry of nutrients and comforting essence. As we delve deeper into its healing embrace, we witness how this humble elixir becomes a conduit for wellness, offering a sanctuary for rejuvenation and restoration.

Close your eyes for a moment and envision a spoonful of blackstrap molasses, dark and velvety, flowing gracefully into a cup of warm water. As you take a sip, a wave of nourishment gently cascades through your body, imbuing you with a sense of vitality and revitalization. Blackstrap molasses becomes the soothing balm that nurtures and replenishes, inviting the whispers of healing to permeate every cell.

Within the pages of this chapter, you will encounter stories of individuals who have experienced profound healing through their encounters with blackstrap molasses. From those who have sought relief from physical ailments to those who have found solace in the nurturing embrace of its sweetness, each story serves as a testament to the power of this elixir to restore balance and harmony.

Blackstrap molasses becomes a faithful ally, supporting us in our pursuit of well-being. Its rich mineral and nutrient content become the building blocks of restoration, nourishing our bodies from within. But it goes beyond the physical realm , it becomes an invitation to tend to our emotional well-being, reminding us of the importance of self-care, self-compassion, and the restoration of our inner landscape.

As we surrender to the whispers of healing, blackstrap molasses becomes a gentle guide, offering us a sanctuary of restoration. It encourages us to listen to the needs of our bodies, to embrace practices that foster vitality, and to create space for healing to unfold. It reminds us that healing is not just a destination but a journey , a continuous dance of nourishment and self-discovery.

As you immerse yourself in the stories and experiences within this chapter, let the whispers of healing envelop you. Allow blackstrap molasses to be your companion on this path of restoration, reminding you that you have the power to cultivate well-being from within. Embrace the practices that nourish your body, mind, and spirit, and let the whispers of healing guide you to a place of vibrant health and vitality.

"Nourishing Secrets: Unveiling the Healing Power of Blackstrap Molasses" becomes more than just a book; it becomes a beacon of hope and a roadmap to wellness. It urges us to honor our bodies and honor the healing journey, recognizing that within us lies the capacity for restoration and renewal. So, dear reader, let blackstrap molasses be the catalyst for your own journey of healing, embracing the whispers of well-being and restoring harmony in your life.

Chapter 12: Blackstrap Molasses and the Dance of Connection: Embracing Love and Unity

[>1000]

In the mesmerizing tapestry of "Nourishing Secrets: Unveiling the Healing Power of Blackstrap Molasses," Chapter 12 weaves a profound narrative of love and unity, revealing the transformative power of blackstrap molasses in fostering deep connections and embracing the beauty of togetherness. Within these heartfelt pages, you will uncover the profound connection between blackstrap molasses and the dance of love, compassion, and the intertwining threads that bind us all.

Imagine a gathering, where souls from all walks of life come together, their hearts beating in unison, their spirits entwined. It is within this sacred space that blackstrap molasses becomes the elixir that fuels the dance of connection , a sweet reminder that we are all interconnected, all part of a greater whole.

In this chapter, we embark on a soul-stirring journey that explores the transformative power of blackstrap molasses in nurturing love and unity , the essence that transcends boundaries, embraces diversity, and celebrates the beauty of our shared humanity. As we delve deeper into its essence, we witness how this humble elixir becomes a catalyst for profound connections, forging bonds that extend far beyond the surface.

Close your eyes for a moment and envision a table adorned with an array of dishes, infused with the warmth and richness of blackstrap molasses. As you partake in the communal feast, a sense of belonging and kinship washes over you , a reminder that love and unity are the true nourishment that sustains us all. Blackstrap molasses becomes the sweet glue that binds hearts, fostering a sense of connection and understanding.

Within the pages of this chapter, you will encounter stories of individuals who have experienced the transformative power of blackstrap molasses in fostering deep connections. From shared meals that transcend language barriers to moments of vulnerability and empathy, each story serves as a testament to the power of this elixir to dissolve boundaries and nurture the bonds of love and unity.

Blackstrap molasses becomes a sacred symbol, a reminder that beneath our external differences, we are all interconnected. Its sweet essence becomes the language of the heart, transcending barriers and bringing us closer together. It becomes an invitation to embrace the richness of diversity, to listen and learn from one another, and to celebrate the beauty that emerges when we stand united.

As we surrender to the dance of connection, blackstrap molasses becomes a guiding light, illuminating the path of love and unity. It urges us to see beyond superficial differences, to extend compassion and kindness to all beings, and to cultivate a sense of belonging in our communities. It reminds us that in the web of life, our actions ripple outward, creating waves of love and unity that have the power to transform the world.

As you immerse yourself in the stories and experiences within this chapter, let the dance of connection envelop you. Allow blackstrap molasses to bc your companion on this journey of love and unity, reminding you of the inherent beauty and interconnectedness of all beings. Embrace the opportunities to forge meaningful connections, to extend a hand of compassion, and to celebrate the diversity that colors our world.

"Nourishing Secrets: Unveiling the Healing Power of Blackstrap Molasses" becomes more than just a book; it becomes a testament to the power of love and unity in creating a harmonious world. It urges us to cherish the connections we share, to foster empathy and understanding, and to recognize that we are all part of a grand symphony of life. So, dear reader, let blackstrap molasses be the catalyst for your own dance of connection, inspiring you to extend love, kindness, and unity to all those you encounter on your journey.

Chapter 13: Blackstrap Molasses and the Path of Resilience: Embracing Strength and Overcoming Challenges [>1000]

Within the captivating narrative of "Nourishing Secrets: Unveiling the Healing Power of Blackstrap Molasses," Chapter 13 emerges as a poignant tale of resilience , a testament to the unwavering strength that lies within each of us when faced with challenges. In these heartfelt pages, you will uncover the profound connection between blackstrap molasses and the transformative journey of embracing our inner fortitude and rising above adversity.

Picture a stormy night, raindrops cascading against the windowpane, the howling wind carrying tales of struggle and perseverance. It is in these moments of darkness that blackstrap molasses becomes the beacon of hope, a sweet reminder that within us resides the power to overcome, to weather the storms of life, and to emerge stronger than ever before.

In this chapter, we embark on a soul-stirring exploration that delves into the transformative power of blackstrap molasses in nurturing resilience , a powerful elixir that fuels our spirit, infusing us with the determination to face life's challenges head-on. As we journey through its essence, we bear witness to the extraordinary stories of individuals who have summoned their inner strength with the aid of blackstrap molasses, forging an unwavering path of resilience.

Close your eyes for a moment and imagine a small bottle of blackstrap molasses, its dark hue radiating an aura of tenacity and fortitude. As you taste its richness, a wave of energy surges through your veins, invigorating your spirit and igniting a fire within. Blackstrap molasses becomes the catalyst that emboldens us, reminding us that even in the face of adversity, we possess an inherent resilience that can carry us through the darkest of times.

Within the pages of this chapter, you will encounter stories of individuals who have overcome immense challenges with the aid of blackstrap molasses. From physical ailments to emotional struggles, each story is a testament to the indomitable human spirit and the power of this humble elixir to nourish not only our bodies but also our souls. It becomes a beacon of hope, illuminating the path of resilience and inspiring us to rise above our circumstances.

Blackstrap molasses becomes a faithful companion, whispering of encouragement and strength in moments of doubt. Its nutritional richness becomes a source of sustenance for our bodies, fueling us with the energy needed to face adversity. But it extends beyond the physical , it becomes a symbol of our ability to endure, to find solace in the face of hardship, and to emerge transformed on the other side.

As we surrender to the path of resilience, blackstrap molasses becomes our guiding light, reminding us that challenges are not obstacles but opportunities for growth. It urges us to tap into our inner wellspring of strength, to cultivate self-compassion, and to trust in our ability to navigate life's twists and turns. It becomes an invitation to embrace our scars as badges of honor, testaments to the battles we have fought and conquered.

As you immerse yourself in the stories and experiences within this chapter, let the path of resilience resonate within you. Allow blackstrap molasses to be your ally on this journey, empowering you to confront challenges with unwavering determination and to emerge stronger and wiser. Embrace the opportunities for growth, knowing that within you lies the capacity to transform adversity into triumph.

"Nourishing Secrets: Unveiling the Healing Power of Blackstrap Molasses" becomes more than just a book; it becomes a testament to the resilience of the human spirit. It urges us to embrace our inner strength, to celebrate our ability to rise above, and to extend compassion and support to others on their own journeys. So, dear reader, let blackstrap molasses be the catalyst for your own path of resilience, reminding you of the unwavering strength that resides within your heart. Embrace the challenges, knowing that they are the

stepping stones that lead you to
greatness.

Chapter 14: Blackstrap Molasses and the Symphony of Gratitude: Embracing the Gift of Appreciation
[>1000]

In the soul-stirring tale of "Nourishing
Secrets: Unveiling the Healing Power
of Blackstrap Molasses," Chapter 14
unfolds as a harmonious symphony of
gratitude , a heartfelt tribute to the
profound power of appreciation and its
transformative effect on our lives.
Within these pages, you will uncover
the profound connection between
blackstrap molasses and the journey of
embracing gratitude, enriching our

lives with the sweet nectar of thankfulness.

Imagine a serene morning, the sun rising gracefully over the horizon, painting the world in hues of gold and amber. It is in these moments of stillness that blackstrap molasses becomes the elixir of gratitude, a gentle reminder to cherish the blessings that grace our lives, both big and small.

In this chapter, we embark on an enchanting exploration that delves into the transformative power of blackstrap molasses in nurturing gratitude , a profound elixir that fills our hearts with appreciation for the wonders that surround us. As we delve deeper into its essence, we witness how this humble elixir becomes a catalyst for a shift in perspective, enriching our lives with the beauty of gratitude.

Close your eyes for a moment and envision a jar of blackstrap molasses, its velvety texture and rich aroma evoking a sense of comfort and joy. As you savor its sweetness, a wave of thankfulness washes over you, illuminating the countless blessings that grace your existence. Blackstrap molasses becomes the catalyst that opens our eyes to the richness of life, urging us to embrace the gift of appreciation.

Within the pages of this chapter, you will encounter stories of individuals who have experienced the profound impact of gratitude with the aid of blackstrap molasses. From moments of simple joy to profound acts of kindness, each story serves as a testament to the power of this elixir to infuse our lives with a sense of wonder and appreciation. It becomes a symphony of gratitude, celebrating the beauty that resides in every aspect of our lives.

Blackstrap molasses becomes a faithful companion on our journey of gratitude, reminding us to pause, to reflect, and to count our blessings. Its sweetness becomes a metaphor for the joys that we often overlook in the hustle of everyday life. It becomes an invitation to savor each moment, to find solace in the little things, and to cultivate a heart brimming with appreciation.

As we surrender to the symphony of gratitude, blackstrap molasses becomes our guiding conductor, leading us on a journey of mindfulness and thankfulness. It urges us to shift our focus from what we lack to the abundance that surrounds us, to express gratitude for the relationships, experiences, and gifts that color our lives. It becomes an invitation to extend gratitude not only to others but also to ourselves , for the resilience we embody, for the love we share, and for the unique journey we traverse.

As you immerse yourself in the stories and experiences within this chapter, let the symphony of gratitude resonate within you. Allow blackstrap molasses to be your ally on this journey, enriching your life with the spirit of appreciation and joy. Embrace the practice of gratitude, knowing that within this simple act lies the key to unlocking a profound sense of contentment and fulfillment.

"Nourishing Secrets: Unveiling the Healing Power of Blackstrap Molasses" becomes more than just a book; it becomes a celebration of gratitude and the joys of living. It urges us to cherish the beauty that exists within and around us, to be present in each moment, and to extend gratitude as a ripple of love into the world. So, dear reader, let blackstrap molasses be the catalyst for your own symphony of gratitude, allowing the sweet notes of appreciation to fill your heart and enrich every facet of your existence.

Chapter 15: Blackstrap Molasses and the Journey of Self-Discovery: Embracing Authenticity and Inner Wisdom
[>1000]

In the captivating tale of "Nourishing Secrets: Unveiling the Healing Power of Blackstrap Molasses," Chapter 15 unfolds as a transformative journey of self-discovery , a profound exploration of embracing authenticity and tapping into our inner wisdom. Within these heartfelt pages, you will uncover the profound connection between blackstrap molasses and the path of self-exploration, empowering us to embrace our true selves and navigate life with grace and authenticity.

Imagine a tranquil evening, the moon casting its gentle glow upon the earth, illuminating the path of self-discovery. It is in these moments of introspection that blackstrap molasses becomes the elixir of self-awareness , a sweet reminder to delve deep into the recesses of our being, uncovering the treasures that lie within.

In this chapter, we embark on an enchanting odyssey that delves into the transformative power of blackstrap molasses in nurturing self-discovery , a potent elixir that ignites the flame of authenticity, guiding us towards a profound understanding of ourselves.

As we venture into its essence, we witness how this humble elixir becomes a catalyst for embracing our unique journey and awakening the dormant wisdom that resides within.

Close your eyes for a moment and envision a cup of blackstrap molasses, its rich aroma and velvety texture inviting you to savor its essence. As you take a sip, a wave of self-acceptance washes over you, embracing every facet of your being , the light and the shadows. Blackstrap molasses becomes the catalyst that empowers us to embrace our true selves, to unravel the layers of conditioning and expectations, and to step into the authenticity that defines us.

Within the pages of this chapter, you will encounter stories of individuals who have embarked on the transformative journey of self-discovery with the aid of blackstrap molasses. From moments of introspection to acts of self-care and empowerment, each story serves as a testament to the power of this elixir to nourish not only our bodies but also our souls. It becomes a compass that guides us towards our true essence, awakening the wisdom that resides within.

Blackstrap molasses becomes a trusted companion, a gentle voice that whispers encouragement and self-compassion. Its depth becomes a mirror that reflects our true selves, reminding us to embrace our strengths, acknowledge our vulnerabilities, and honor the unique path we tread. It becomes an invitation to listen to the whispers of our hearts, to honor our passions and desires, and to live authentically, unapologetically.

As we surrender to the journey of self-discovery, blackstrap molasses becomes our guiding light, illuminating the path of inner wisdom and self-acceptance. It urges us to cultivate self-love, to trust our intuition, and to honor our truth. It becomes an invitation to shed the masks we wear, to release the expectations of others, and to embrace the freedom that comes with living in alignment with our authentic selves.

As you immerse yourself in the stories and experiences within this chapter, let the journey of self-discovery resonate within you. Allow blackstrap molasses to be your ally on this transformative path, empowering you to embrace your true essence and to navigate life with grace and authenticity. Embrace the opportunities for self-reflection, knowing that within this exploration lies the key to unlocking your fullest potential.

"Nourishing Secrets: Unveiling the Healing Power of Blackstrap Molasses" becomes more than just a book; it becomes a guidebook for the journey of self-discovery. It urges us to embark on the quest to know ourselves deeply, to celebrate our uniqueness, and to honor the wisdom that resides within. So, dear reader, let blackstrap molasses be the catalyst for your own voyage of self-discovery, allowing your authentic self to shine brightly and illuminate the world.

Printed in Great Britain
by Amazon

44317169R00040